EBV & Autoimmune Disease

A Beginner's Guide to Understanding Epstein-Barr Virus and Its Link to Autoimmune Conditions

mf

copyright © 2025 Jeffrey Winzant

All rights reserved No part of this book may be reproduced, or stored in a retrieval system, or transmitted in any form or by any means, electronic, mechanical, photocopying, recording, or otherwise, without express written permission of the publisher.

Disclaimer

By reading this disclaimer, you are accepting the terms of the disclaimer in full. If you disagree with this disclaimer, please do not read the guide.

All of the content within this guide is provided for informational and educational purposes only, and should not be accepted as independent medical or other professional advice. The author is not a doctor, physician, nurse, mental health provider, or registered nutritionist/dietician. Therefore, using and reading this guide does not establish any form of a physician-patient relationship.

Always consult with a physician or another qualified health provider with any issues or questions you might have regarding any sort of medical condition. Do not ever disregard any qualified professional medical advice or delay seeking that advice because of anything you have read in this guide. The information in this guide is not intended to be any sort of medical advice and should not be used in lieu of any medical advice by a licensed and qualified medical professional.

The information in this guide has been compiled from a variety of known sources. However, the author cannot attest to or guarantee the accuracy of each source and thus should not be held liable for any errors or omissions.

You acknowledge that the publisher of this guide will not be held liable for any loss or damage of any kind incurred as a result of this guide or the reliance on any information provided within this guide. You acknowledge and agree that you assume all risk and responsibility for any action you undertake in response to the information in this guide.

Using this guide does not guarantee any particular result (e.g., weight loss or a cure). By reading this guide, you acknowledge that there are no guarantees to any specific outcome or results you can expect.

All product names, diet plans, or names used in this guide are for identification purposes only and are the property of their respective owners. The use of these names does not imply endorsement. All other trademarks cited herein are the property of their respective owners.

Where applicable, this guide is not intended to be a substitute for the original work of this diet plan and is, at most, a supplement to the original work for this diet plan and never a direct substitute. This guide is a personal expression of the facts of that diet plan.

Where applicable, persons shown in the cover images are stock photography models and the publisher has obtained the rights to use the images through license agreements with third-party stock image companies.

Table of Contents

Introduction   7
The Hidden Connection Between EBV & Autoimmune Disease   10
   Why So Many People with Autoimmune Disorders Also Have EBV   10
   The Science Behind EBV Reactivation and Immune Dysfunction   13
What Is Epstein-Barr Virus (EBV)?   17
   How EBV Infects the Body and Stays Dormant   17
   EBV Reactivation: What Triggers It?   19
   The Difference Between Acute EBV, Chronic EBV, and Reactivated EBV   23
The Link Between EBV and Autoimmune Diseases   26
   How EBV Can Confuse and Attack the Immune System   26
   Autoimmune Conditions Most Commonly Linked to EBV   28
   Can EBV Be the Root Cause of Autoimmune Disease?   31
Recognizing the Symptoms of EBV & Autoimmune Flares   33
   How to Tell the Difference Between EBV Symptoms and Autoimmune Symptoms   33
   Common Overlapping Symptoms   34
   When to Get Tested for EBV and Autoimmune Markers   37
Triggers that Worsen EBV and Autoimmune Conditions   40
   The Role of Stress and Cortisol in EBV Reactivation   40
   How Gut Health & Leaky Gut Make Autoimmune Symptoms Worse   41
   The Impact of Diet, Sugar, and Processed Foods   43
   Sleep, Toxins, and Other Environmental Triggers   44
Supporting Your Immune System When Living with EBV & Autoimmune Disease   46
   How to Reduce Inflammation and Minimize Symptom Flares   46

    The Role of Nutrition in Managing EBV and Autoimmunity 47
    The Importance of Rest, Gentle Movement, and Mindfulness 49
    Should You Take Supplements? What the Science Says   50

Navigating Medical & Holistic Approaches   53
    What Conventional Medicine Says About EBV & Autoimmune Disease   53
    Alternative & Holistic Approaches to Managing EBV   55
    Blood Tests and Markers to Request from Your Doctor   56
    Working with an Integrative Health Practitioner   58

Long-Term Strategies for Managing EBV & Autoimmune Symptoms   60
    Lifestyle Adjustments That Reduce Autoimmune Flares   60
    How to Prevent EBV Reactivation in the Future   68
    Emotional and Mental Health: Coping with a Chronic Condition   75
    Creating a Personalized Health Plan That Works for You   77

Conclusion   80
FAQs   84
References and Helpful Links   87

Introduction

Epstein-Barr Virus (EBV) is one of the most common viruses worldwide, with an estimated 90% of the global population infected at some point in their lives. Epstein-Barr Virus (EBV), part of the herpesvirus family, is commonly transmitted via saliva and close interpersonal interactions.

It is best known for causing infectious mononucleosis, or "mono," often referred to as the "kissing disease." For most individuals, an EBV infection resolves without major complications. However, its long-term implications are far from fully understood.

Recent research has pointed to potential connections between EBV and the development of various autoimmune diseases. Autoimmune conditions, such as multiple sclerosis, systemic lupus erythematosus, and rheumatoid arthritis, occur when the immune system mistakenly attacks the body's own tissues.

Scientists have observed patterns suggesting that EBV might act as a triggering or contributing factor for these diseases. While the exact mechanisms remain under study, theories include the virus's ability to alter immune system function, persist in the body long after the initial infection, and possibly mimic proteins found in human tissues.

Understanding the relationship between EBV and autoimmune disorders is critical for advancing medical knowledge. This connection could help explain why some individuals develop autoimmune conditions while others do not. It also opens the door for further scientific exploration into how latent viral infections might influence long-term health.

In this guide, we will talk about the following:

- The Hidden Connection Between EBV & Autoimmune Disease
- What is Epstein-Barr Virus (EBV)?
- The Link Between EBV and Autoimmune Diseases
- Recognizing the Symptoms of EBV & Autoimmune Flares
- Triggers That Worsen EBV and Autoimmune Conditions
- Supporting Your Immune System When Living with EBV & Autoimmune Disease
- Navigating Medical & Holistic Approaches
- Long-Term Strategies for Managing EBV & Autoimmune Symptoms

Keep reading to learn more about EBV and its potential impact on autoimmune diseases. By the end, you will have a better understanding of how this virus plays a role in the development and management of these conditions.

The Hidden Connection Between EBV & Autoimmune Disease

The Epstein-Barr Virus (EBV) is one of the most common viruses in the world. Most people encounter EBV at some point in their lives, often without even realizing it. For many, it causes little to no trouble.

However, for some people, EBV can lead to long-term health complications, especially when it comes to autoimmune diseases. This chapter will explore why so many individuals with autoimmune disorders also have EBV and explain the role EBV plays in triggering immune system problems.

Why So Many People with Autoimmune Disorders Also Have EBV

Studies reveal a striking overlap between autoimmune diseases and previous EBV infections. Once someone contracts EBV, the virus remains in their body for life, typically in a dormant state. For many, this latency causes no further issues.

However, people with autoimmune conditions often exhibit signs that EBV has been much more active in their systems, raising the question of whether a deeper connection exists.

EBV Stays in the Body Permanently

Once EBV infects someone, it never fully leaves their body. Instead, the virus embeds itself within certain cells of the immune system, called B-lymphocytes, or B cells. These cells play a key role in human immunity by producing antibodies to fight infections. EBV's ability to insert itself into these cells gives it a long-lasting presence.

While dormant EBV typically goes unnoticed, it can "wake up" or reactivate under specific conditions, such as stress or illness. When this happens, the dormant virus begins replicating, which may result in symptoms or immune system confusion. This potential for reactivation is significant for people with autoimmune diseases, as it can worsen their immune dysfunction.

EBV Can Trigger Autoimmune Problems

Much of the evidence linking EBV to autoimmune disease comes from its ability to interfere with the immune system. One well-documented phenomenon is called "molecular mimicry." This occurs when proteins on the surface of EBV resemble proteins naturally found in the body's tissues.

The immune system, attempting to attack the virus, may be "tricked" into also attacking healthy cells and proteins that closely resemble EBV. Over time, this misdirected immune response can lead to systemic inflammation and autoimmunity.

Additionally, EBV creates further complications by altering the behavior of B cells. Its presence can stimulate these cells to behave abnormally, contributing to the production of harmful autoantibodies. These autoantibodies mistakenly target and damage the body's own tissues, exacerbating autoimmune diseases like lupus or rheumatoid arthritis.

Some People Are Genetically More Vulnerable

Genetics plays an important role in explaining why not everyone with EBV develops an autoimmune disease. Specific genetic profiles may make certain individuals more susceptible to autoimmune conditions when confronted with immune stressors such as viral infections.

Genes that influence the immune system, particularly those regulating the inflammatory response, appear to interact with EBV in ways that increase the likelihood of autoimmunity.

Researchers continue to explore these genetic factors, as understanding which individuals are most vulnerable could help identify at-risk populations and lead to earlier interventions.

The Science Behind EBV Reactivation and Immune Dysfunction

To understand how EBV contributes to autoimmune diseases, it's crucial to examine its behavior within the body and its interaction with the immune system. The virus has developed sophisticated strategies to evade detection and manipulate the body's defenses, which can lead to immune dysfunction over time.

How EBV Reactivates

After its initial infection, EBV typically enters a dormant phase, where it remains inactive within its host cells. However, under certain conditions, the virus can reactivate. Several factors may create the conditions necessary for reactivation, including the following:

1. *Stress:* Chronic or severe stress can weaken the immune system, creating an opportunity for EBV to reactivate. Stress impacts the body by increasing levels of cortisol, a hormone that can dampen immune activity and leave the system more vulnerable to latent viruses.
2. *Other Illnesses:* When the immune system becomes preoccupied with fighting another infection, it may

have fewer resources available to suppress EBV. This allows the virus to replicate and regain activity.
3. ***Lifestyle Factors:*** Lack of sleep, poor diet, or exposure to toxins can all contribute to general immune strain, which may lower the body's defenses and lead to EBV reactivation.

When the virus reactivates, it begins producing viral proteins and viral particles, which the immune system recognizes as foreign. This recognition sparks an immune response that can lead to widespread inflammation and immune imbalance.

The Impact on the Immune System

EBV directly disrupts multiple aspects of the immune system, compounding the confusion and inflammation that characterize autoimmune diseases. Two major consequences of EBV reactivation are chronic immune activation and T-cell exhaustion.

1. ***Chronic Immune Activation:*** During reactivation, EBV creates an inflammatory environment within the body. It stimulates the release of cytokines, which are signaling molecules that ramp up the immune response. While these molecules are useful for combating infections, their prolonged presence can lead to excessive inflammation. Chronic inflammation is a hallmark of autoimmune diseases like lupus and rheumatoid arthritis.

2. ***T-Cell Exhaustion:*** T cells are another critical component of the immune system, responsible for attacking infected or abnormal cells. EBV can interfere with T-cell function over time, leading to a state known as T-cell exhaustion. This leaves the immune system less effective at controlling EBV and other threats, further disrupting immune regulation and increasing the risk of autoimmune responses.

Long-Term Immune Dysfunction

Over time, repeated cycles of EBV reactivation and immune suppression can have a cumulative effect on the body. Persistent inflammation and immune dysregulation may wear down the immune system's ability to maintain balance, contributing to the progression of autoimmune diseases.

Additionally, EBV has been observed to affect the communication between immune cells. It alters the signals that help immune cells coordinate their activity, which can create confusion within the system. These changes further compound the difficulty of distinguishing between healthy tissue and harmful invaders, reinforcing the autoimmune process.

Research and Future Directions

Ongoing research continues to shed light on the mechanisms through which EBV influences immune dysfunction. Scientists are investigating how factors like co-infections, environmental exposures, and genetic predispositions amplify the relationship between EBV and autoimmunity. Such studies hold the potential for developing interventions that target EBV's impact on the immune system.

The connection between EBV and autoimmune diseases represents a growing area of interest for medical professionals and researchers. EBV's ability to reappear decades after its initial infection and disrupt the immune system presents unique challenges. While not all individuals with EBV go on to develop autoimmune conditions, the virus's role as a potential trigger or contributor is becoming harder to ignore.

By understanding how EBV influences the immune system, researchers hope to pave the way for future breakthroughs in treating and potentially preventing autoimmune diseases.

What Is Epstein-Barr Virus (EBV)?

The Epstein-Barr Virus (EBV) is one of the most common viruses, affecting millions of people worldwide. Discovered in 1964 by Dr. Michael Epstein and Dr. Yvonne Barr, the virus was first identified in samples from individuals with Burkitt's lymphoma, a type of cancer.

Part of the herpesvirus family, EBV is also known as human herpesvirus 4 (HHV-4). It is highly contagious and often transmitted through saliva, earning it the nickname "the kissing disease." The virus primarily targets B cells—a type of white blood cell responsible for producing antibodies that help the body combat infections.

How EBV Infects the Body and Stays Dormant

EBV spreads primarily through bodily fluids, particularly saliva. This is why it is sometimes referred to as the "kissing disease," as it is frequently transmitted through close personal contact or sharing utensils.

Once it enters the body, EBV travels through the mucous membranes of the throat or nose and targets B-lymphocytes, a type of white blood cell involved in the immune response.

After infecting the host, EBV goes through two key phases:

1. **Primary Infection**

   The first encounter with EBV, known as the primary infection, typically involves the active replication of the virus. During this phase, EBV targets specific cells in the body, including epithelial cells in the mucous membranes of the throat and B-lymphocytes, or "B cells," which are a type of white blood cell that plays a key role in the immune system.

   The symptoms of primary EBV infection vary significantly from person to person. For some, the infection appears as a mild, flu-like illness with little cause for concern. However, for others, the primary infection manifests as infectious mononucleosis, often shortened to "mono."

   Infectious mononucleosis, most common in teenagers and young adults, is marked by symptoms such as extreme fatigue, fever, a sore throat, swollen lymph nodes, and an enlarged spleen. These symptoms might last a few weeks to months before the virus enters the next phase.

2. **Latency**

After the body successfully controls the initial EBV infection, the virus does not leave the body completely. Instead, it enters a dormant state known as "latency." During this phase, EBV resides quietly within B cells and certain tissues, where it produces minimal proteins. This minimal activity allows EBV to effectively avoid detection by the immune system, remaining hidden.

For most people, latent EBV remains silent for the rest of their lives and causes no further complications. The immune system monitors the virus and keeps it from becoming active again. However, EBV's dormant state is essentially a waiting game. Under specific conditions that weaken the immune system or create stress within the body, the virus can reactivate, leading to potential health consequences.

EBV Reactivation: What Triggers It?

EBV reactivation occurs when the virus transitions from its dormant state back into active replication. This process allows the production of new viral particles, which can sometimes lead to noticeable symptoms and potentially impact overall health.

Many people with EBV reactivation remain asymptomatic, meaning they experience no apparent signs of illness. Others, however, may develop health complications, especially if their immune system is weakened.

Understanding what triggers EBV reactivation is crucial in identifying why some people are more affected by the virus in its later stages. While the reasons for reactivation can vary widely, several key factors have been identified as potential triggers.

1. **Stress**

    Stress is one of the most commonly documented triggers for EBV reactivation. When the body undergoes significant physical or emotional stress, it releases higher levels of a hormone called cortisol.

    While cortisol is helpful in small amounts, chronic or severe stress can suppress the immune system's ability to function fully. A weakened immune response gives EBV the opportunity to replicate and reactivate, allowing the virus to awaken from its dormant state.

    Examples of stressors that may contribute to EBV reactivation include:

    - Prolonged work-related or personal stress
    - Recovery from surgery or major injury
    - Intense physical exertion without proper recovery

2. Immune Suppression

Conditions or treatments that suppress the immune system significantly increase the risk of EBV reactivation. For example:

Individuals undergoing chemotherapy or taking immunosuppressive medications for autoimmune diseases may have reduced immune activity, enabling EBV to reactivate.

Diseases like HIV/AIDS, which directly weaken immune defenses, can also make reactivation more likely.

When the immune system cannot maintain control over dormant viruses, EBV is among those that reactivate and potentially worsen health outcomes.

3. Hormonal Changes

Hormonal shifts are another possible trigger. Hormonal changes associated with puberty, pregnancy, or menopause may disrupt the body's typical processes enough to provide a window for EBV to reactivate. While research into the exact mechanisms is ongoing, hormonal fluctuations are believed to affect immune system function and create conditions that support viral activity.

4. **Co-Infections**

   EBV is not the only infection that puts stress on the immune system. People recovering from illnesses such as the flu, Lyme disease, or bacterial infections may face additional strain on their immune defenses.

   When the immune system is occupied fighting other infections, it may leave EBV unchecked, allowing reactivation to occur. The more severe the co-infection, the greater the likelihood of EBV's re-emergence.

5. **Poor Sleep and Diet**

   Lifestyle factors such as inadequate sleep, malnutrition, or a lack of essential nutrients can also weaken the body's ability to keep EBV dormant. Regular sleep is vital for immune repair and recovery, while diet directly influences the body's ability to produce effective immune cells. When these factors are impaired, EBV may find an opportunity to reactivate, and its impact on health could become more noticeable.

It's important to note that not everyone exposed to these triggers will experience EBV reactivation. The immune system's effectiveness varies from person to person, influenced by genetic makeup, overall health, and other individual factors. Additionally, the severity of EBV reactivation can differ widely, ranging from mild symptoms to significant health complications.

People with strong and well-regulated immune systems may experience little to no impact from EBV reactivation, while those with underlying immune challenges may face more pronounced health effects.

The Difference Between Acute EBV, Chronic EBV, and Reactivated EBV

When discussing EBV-related health conditions, it's essential to understand the distinctions between acute infection, chronic infection, and reactivation. These terms describe different stages or manifestations of the virus.

Acute EBV Infection

This is the initial phase of the virus after someone is first exposed. Acute EBV infection commonly presents with symptoms of infectious mononucleosis, such as severe fatigue, fever, a sore throat, and enlarged lymph nodes. These symptoms usually resolve within 2–4 weeks and the individual moves into the latent stage.

Chronic EBV

This term refers to a rare condition where EBV remains **active in the body for an extended period**, continuing to replicate and cause symptoms. Chronic Active EBV

(CAEBV) is characterized by persistent fever, swollen lymph nodes, and organ damage, and it requires medical attention.

It's important to note that most people with EBV do not develop a chronic infection, and chronic EBV should not be confused with the general presence of the virus in its dormant state.

Reactivated EBV

When the virus wakes from dormancy, it is considered reactivated. This can happen years or even decades after the initial infection. Reactivation may **occur without noticeable symptoms**, or it may lead to overlapping symptoms such as fatigue, muscle pain, and low-grade fever. Reactivated EBV can sometimes exacerbate existing health conditions, particularly autoimmune diseases.

Understanding these phases can help distinguish between primary infection, dormant, and active states of the virus in relation to overall health.

EBV is a widespread virus that infects most people at some point in their lives, often remaining silent in a dormant state after the initial infection. However, under certain conditions, it can reactivate and potentially contribute to a range of health challenges.

Recognizing the triggers and differences between acute, chronic, and reactivated EBV provides crucial context for understanding how EBV interacts with the human immune system, setting the foundation for its potential links to other medical conditions.

The Link Between EBV and Autoimmune Diseases

Epstein-Barr Virus (EBV) has long been associated with various autoimmune diseases, raising questions about whether it plays a role in triggering or exacerbating these conditions. To understand this connection, it's important to explore how EBV interacts with the immune system and the specific autoimmune conditions most commonly linked with the virus. This chapter will also look at whether EBV might be a root cause of autoimmunity or simply one of many contributing factors.

How EBV Can Confuse and Attack the Immune System

EBV is known for its ability to manipulate and disrupt the immune system, which can lead to long-lasting consequences. After the initial infection, the virus remains dormant in the immune system, specifically within B cells. These cells are crucial for fighting infections and maintaining immune balance. However, EBV's presence in these cells can interfere with their normal function.

Immune Confusion and Molecular Mimicry

One way EBV confuses the immune system is through a process called molecular mimicry. This means that certain proteins produced by EBV look very similar to proteins found naturally in the body.

> When the immune system tries to attack the virus, it might accidentally target the body's own tissues, mistaking them for EBV. Over time, this mix-up can cause the immune system to turn against the body, resulting in autoimmune diseases.

Chronic Activation and Immune Dysregulation

EBV also keeps the immune system in a heightened state of alert. Even when the virus is dormant, small amounts of viral proteins may be expressed, continuing to stimulate the immune system. This persistent activation can lead to chronic inflammation, a key feature of many autoimmune conditions.

> Additionally, EBV can affect communication between immune cells, disrupting their ability to coordinate a proper response. These disruptions further increase the risk of autoimmunity by creating an environment where the immune system struggles to differentiate between harmful agents and healthy tissues.

T-Cell Exhaustion

Another impact of EBV is its ability to weaken T cells, another type of immune cell that plays a major role in identifying and killing infected cells. Frequent or prolonged battles with EBV can cause these immune cells to become "exhausted," making it harder for the body to keep the virus under control. This weakened immune response can contribute to autoimmune disease by creating conditions where EBV can reactivate and further disrupt immune regulation.

Autoimmune Conditions Most Commonly Linked to EBV

EBV has been associated with several autoimmune diseases. Each condition has its own set of symptoms and affects different parts of the body, but they often share similar underlying immune dysfunctions. Here are some of the autoimmune diseases most closely linked to EBV.

1. **Hashimoto's Thyroiditis**

    Hashimoto's thyroiditis is an autoimmune condition that attacks the thyroid, a gland responsible for regulating metabolism, energy, and many other bodily functions. Researchers suspect a link between EBV and Hashimoto's because the virus can trigger inflammation in the thyroid gland.

This inflammation might set off an immune response where the body starts attacking its own thyroid tissues. People with Hashimoto's often experience symptoms such as fatigue, weight gain, and cold sensitivity.

2. Lupus

Lupus is a systemic autoimmune disease that causes the immune system to attack multiple organs, such as the skin, kidneys, and joints. Studies suggest that individuals with lupus may have a higher rate of prior EBV infection compared to the general population.

EBV's ability to manipulate the immune system, particularly through molecular mimicry, is thought to play a role in the development of lupus. For example, EBV proteins might resemble normal cell components, leading the immune system to mistakenly attack healthy cells.

3. Multiple Sclerosis (MS)

Multiple sclerosis is a neurological condition where the immune system damages the protective covering of nerves, known as myelin. A strong connection between EBV and MS has been observed in scientific studies.

Nearly all individuals with MS have been infected with EBV at some point in their lives. One theory is that EBV reactivation in the brain triggers inflammation and abnormal immune responses, contributing to the nerve damage seen in MS.

4. **Rheumatoid Arthritis (RA)**

Rheumatoid arthritis is an autoimmune disease that primarily affects the joints, causing pain, swelling, and stiffness. While the exact cause of RA is unknown, some studies have found higher levels of EBV-related antibodies in people with RA.

This suggests that prior EBV infection may influence the development of the disease. It's possible that EBV contributes to the formation of autoantibodies, molecules that attack the body's own tissues, which is a hallmark of RA.

5. **Sjögren's Syndrome**

Sjögren's syndrome is an autoimmune condition that mainly targets the glands that produce saliva and tears, leading to dry mouth and dry eyes. Evidence suggests that EBV may be involved in disrupting normal gland function in people with Sjögren's syndrome. The virus's presence in certain tissues could trigger immune confusion, leading to chronic inflammation and damage to the glands.

Can EBV Be the Root Cause of Autoimmune Disease?

The idea that EBV could be a root cause of autoimmune disease is still a topic of debate among researchers. While many studies have found strong links between EBV and autoimmunity, it's important to understand that EBV is likely one of many factors involved. Autoimmune diseases are complex and usually result from a combination of genetic, environmental, and immune system factors.

1. **Genetic Predisposition and EBV**

    Genetics plays a significant role in determining whether a person develops an autoimmune disease. Certain genes make individuals more likely to have an overactive or improperly regulated immune system. For people with these genetic risks, EBV may act as a trigger by adding extra stress to an already vulnerable immune system.

2. **EBV as a Catalyst, Not the Sole Cause**

    EBV may not cause autoimmune disease on its own but could act as a catalyst. For instance, someone with a genetic predisposition might remain healthy until encountering specific triggers, such as an EBV infection, chronic stress, or exposure to certain toxins. EBV could exacerbate existing risk factors or tip the balance toward autoimmunity.

3. **Not Everyone with EBV Develops Autoimmunity**

   It's important to note that while EBV is extremely common, not everyone who has been infected with the virus develops an autoimmune disease. Most people carry EBV without experiencing significant health problems. This reinforces the idea that other factors, including genetics and lifestyle, play a role in determining whether EBV contributes to autoimmunity.

The relationship between EBV and autoimmune diseases is complex and multifaceted. While EBV has significant potential to disrupt immune function and contribute to the development of autoimmunity, it is likely just one piece of a larger puzzle. By continuing to study this connection, scientists and healthcare providers hope to uncover more about how autoimmune diseases begin and how they can be managed effectively.

Recognizing the Symptoms of EBV & Autoimmune Flares

The symptoms of Epstein-Barr Virus (EBV) and autoimmune diseases can often overlap, making it difficult to tell one condition from the other. Many people experience similar signs such as fatigue, pain, and inflammation, whether the cause is EBV reactivation, an autoimmune flare, or both.

Understanding the differences and similarities between these symptoms is key to recognizing what might be happening in your body. This chapter explains how to identify these symptoms, highlights the most common ones, and discusses when it might be appropriate to get tested.

How to Tell the Difference Between EBV Symptoms and Autoimmune Symptoms

Distinguishing EBV symptoms from autoimmune symptoms can be tricky since both conditions may provoke similar responses in the body. However, there are key differences to consider. EBV, as a viral infection, primarily triggers short-lived symptoms during reactivation or acute infection.

These may include sore throat, swollen lymph nodes, fever, and fatigue. Such symptoms typically appear suddenly and resolve as the immune system suppresses the viral activity.

Autoimmune symptoms, by contrast, tend to build gradually or persist over extended periods. They often reflect chronic inflammation or immune dysfunction rather than a transient infection. For example, joint pain or organ-specific complications caused by autoimmune conditions like lupus or rheumatoid arthritis might worsen over weeks or months, and flares can be triggered by factors like stress or environmental stimuli.

That said, it is possible for EBV to exacerbate autoimmune symptoms. Reactivation of EBV may act as a trigger, presenting overlapping signs like fatigue or swelling, which can confuse diagnosis. Tracking symptom patterns and duration may help discern whether the underlying cause is viral or autoimmune-related. Consulting a healthcare provider for detailed evaluation often becomes vital in cases of persistent or ambiguous symptoms.

Common Overlapping Symptoms

Some symptoms are common to both EBV and autoimmune conditions, which can make diagnosis difficult. These overlapping symptoms include fatigue, brain fog, joint and muscle pain, and inflammation. Here's a closer look at each:

1. **Chronic Fatigue**

   Fatigue is one of the most common signs of both EBV reactivation and autoimmune disease. However, the nature of the fatigue may vary. Fatigue caused by EBV reactivation is often sudden and overwhelming, leaving you feeling like even basic tasks take immense effort. This kind of tiredness may not improve much with rest.

   Fatigue from an autoimmune condition, on the other hand, is often chronic and comes with other hallmark symptoms of inflammation. For instance, people with conditions like rheumatoid arthritis may feel stiff, heavy, and tired all at once.

2. **Brain Fog**

   Both EBV and autoimmune diseases can cause cognitive issues, often referred to as "brain fog." This includes problems with memory, focus, and mental clarity. Brain fog from EBV reactivation tends to appear gradually and is often accompanied by other physical symptoms such as fatigue or flu-like feelings.

   For autoimmune diseases, brain fog might be more closely related to inflammation or other physical symptoms, such as extreme exhaustion or pain. Many people with autoimmune diseases report that brain fog becomes worse during flares.

3. **Joint & Muscle Pain**

   Pain in the joints and muscles is another symptom that EBV and autoimmune diseases share. During EBV reactivation, muscle and joint pain might resemble soreness caused by a viral infection and is usually accompanied by other signs like fever or swollen lymph nodes. This pain is temporary and often subsides as the immune system brings the virus under control.

   Joint and muscle pain from autoimmune diseases is often more persistent and inflammatory in nature. For example, in rheumatoid arthritis, the joints might feel warm, swollen, or stiff, especially in the morning. Similarly, muscle pain in conditions like lupus may come with other systemic symptoms such as skin rashes or sensitivity to sunlight.

4. **Inflammation & Swelling**

   Inflammation and swelling are key features of many autoimmune conditions, as they often occur due to the immune system's response to perceived threats. Autoimmune-related inflammation may target specific areas, such as the joints in rheumatoid arthritis or the thyroid gland in Hashimoto's thyroiditis.

   EBV, meanwhile, can cause inflammation as well, particularly during its active or reactivated phases.

Swelling of the lymph nodes, along with tenderness, is a classic symptom of EBV-related inflammation. While this inflammation can feel similar to that of autoimmunity, it often has distinguishing symptoms like a sore throat or fever.

When to Get Tested for EBV and Autoimmune Markers

Given the overlap in symptoms, testing can be an essential step in determining whether a person's health issues are caused by EBV, an autoimmune condition, or both.

While general symptoms like fatigue and joint pain may suggest a problem, testing provides more clarity. Here are some indications for seeking medical tests:

1. **Persistent or Severe Symptoms**

    If fatigue, brain fog, pain, or inflammation persist for weeks or months without improvement, it could warrant testing for both EBV and autoimmune markers. Severe or worsening symptoms, such as ongoing fever, unrelieved joint pain, or substantial difficulty performing daily tasks, are also reasons to consult a healthcare professional.

2. **Overlapping Symptoms Without a Clear Cause**

    When symptoms clearly align with one or more conditions but lack a clear explanation, doctors may order tests for EBV antibodies as well as autoimmune markers like antinuclear antibodies (ANA). This is especially relevant if a person has had multiple unexplained instances of illness or chronic inflammation.

3. **Family History or Increased Risk Factors**

   Individuals with a family history of autoimmune disease may have a higher risk of developing autoimmune conditions themselves, especially if they also have a history of EBV infection. Testing may help identify any emerging issues earlier on.

4. **Situations Where Testing Is Recommended**

   Doctors may recommend checking for EBV reactivation through blood tests that look for specific antibodies indicating the presence of an active or recent infection. To identify autoimmune conditions, various markers can be tested, depending on the suspected disease. For example, rheumatoid factor is tested for RA, while thyroid antibodies could confirm Hashimoto's thyroiditis.

   Early testing and diagnosis can help clarify the root causes of overlapping symptoms, setting the groundwork for future care tailored to an individual's health needs.

Understanding how EBV and autoimmune symptoms overlap makes it easier to recognize the underlying issues affecting health. While the symptoms can be complex and sometimes hard to distinguish, testing and further diagnostic efforts can help provide clarity. The next chapters will explore the specific triggers that can worsen these symptoms and what studies reveal about managing related conditions.

Triggers that Worsen EBV and Autoimmune Conditions

Recognizing the triggers that exacerbate symptoms of Epstein-Barr Virus (EBV) and autoimmune diseases is essential for understanding how these conditions affect the body. While these triggers are not direct causes of disease, they can worsen symptoms or make flare-ups more frequent.

This chapter focuses on four major factors that contribute to symptom aggravation: stress and cortisol, gut health, diet and processed foods, and environmental triggers.

The Role of Stress and Cortisol in EBV Reactivation

Stress is one of the most significant factors that can trigger EBV reactivation and worsen autoimmune diseases. When you experience stress, your body releases a hormone called cortisol, which helps you respond to immediate challenges. While this response is useful in small doses, chronic stress can overwhelm the body and have lasting effects on the immune system.

How Stress Affects the Immune System

High levels of cortisol over long periods can suppress the immune system's ability to function properly. This weakened state gives EBV an opportunity to reactivate. The virus takes advantage of a compromised immune system by replicating more easily, which can lead to symptoms such as fatigue, inflammation, and swollen lymph nodes.

For people with autoimmune diseases, stress contributes to immune system imbalance. It increases inflammation, which can lead to flare-ups or worsen existing symptoms. Stress may also interfere with how the body identifies "self" from "non-self," making autoimmune attacks more likely.

The Vicious Cycle of Stress and Symptoms

Stress and symptoms are often part of a cycle. The physical symptoms brought on by EBV or autoimmunity, such as pain or fatigue, can increase emotional stress. This, in turn, leads to a rise in cortisol levels, which may further aggravate the symptoms. Breaking this cycle is crucial, although challenging, for individuals dealing with these conditions.

How Gut Health & Leaky Gut Make Autoimmune Symptoms Worse

The gut is a critical part of overall health and plays a surprising role in both EBV and autoimmune diseases. The term "leaky gut" refers to a condition where the intestinal lining becomes more permeable than it should be, allowing substances that shouldn't normally pass through to enter the bloodstream.

The Gut-Immune System Connection

The gut houses a large portion of the immune system, known as gut-associated lymphoid tissue (GALT). This is the body's first line of defense against harmful bacteria, viruses, and toxins. However, when the gut is unhealthy, it can miscommunicate with the immune system, leading to an overactive or improperly regulated response.

For people with autoimmune diseases, a leaky gut can worsen symptoms by increasing overall inflammation. Tiny particles that leak through the intestinal lining can trigger the immune system to attack, creating a heightened state of immune alertness. If EBV is present in the body, this inflammation provides a fertile ground for the virus to become more active.

Factors Contributing to Poor Gut Health

Certain factors make gut health worse and may lead to or intensify a leaky gut. These include diets high in processed foods, stress, and infections like EBV. When the gut barrier becomes compromised, it sets off a chain reaction of immune dysfunction that can exacerbate autoimmune symptoms and increase the chances of EBV reactivation.

The Impact of Diet, Sugar, and Processed Foods

What you eat plays a major role in your body's ability to manage both EBV and autoimmune conditions. While specific dietary triggers can vary from person to person, research shows that certain foods and eating patterns are linked to increased inflammation and immune dysfunction.

How Processed Foods Affect the Immune System

Processed foods often contain:

- Artificial additives
- Preservatives
- High levels of sugar
- Saturated fats

These substances can fuel inflammation, impair immune function, and disrupt healthy gut bacteria. For individuals dealing with autoimmune conditions, even small amounts of these foods may lead to symptom flare-ups. High sugar intake, in particular, can spike inflammation, reduce immunity, and provide energy for viruses, including EBV, to replicate.

Nutritional Deficiency as a Trigger

Diets that lack essential nutrients, like vitamins D and B, zinc, or omega-3 fatty acids, can weaken the immune system over time. A weakened immune system is less effective at controlling EBV and can contribute to worsening autoimmune symptoms. For example, lack of omega-3 fatty acids, often found in processed and fast foods, is linked to higher levels of inflammation.

Sleep, Toxins, and Other Environmental Triggers

Environmental factors, including poor sleep, exposure to toxins, and other external triggers, also play a role in worsening symptoms of EBV and autoimmune diseases.

The Importance of Sleep for Immune Health

Sleep is one of the body's most powerful tools for maintaining a healthy immune system. During sleep, the immune system undergoes repair and restoration. For those with EBV or autoimmunity, lack of sleep can lead to a more dysregulated immune response. Chronic poor sleep is linked to increased inflammation, making flare-ups more likely.

For instance, people who don't get enough sleep might notice worsening fatigue, increased brain fog, and heightened joint pain. Sleep also affects stress levels by regulating cortisol, meaning poor sleep and high stress often go hand-in-hand in further aggravating symptoms.

Toxins and Immune Dysfunction

Environmental toxins, such as heavy metals, pesticides, or pollutants, can disrupt the immune system and increase the likelihood of EBV reactivation. These toxins may accumulate in the body over time, particularly in organs like the liver, which is responsible for filtration and detoxification.

Autoimmune diseases can also become more severe when the body is exposed to toxins because they add stress to the body's already overburdened immune system. For example, some people report increased joint pain or fatigue when exposed to mold, air pollution, or chemical cleaners.

Other Environmental Triggers

- *Seasonal changes* like colder weather might unbalance the immune system, particularly for people with autoimmune diseases.
- *Viruses and infections* other than EBV may put extra strain on the immune system, making existing symptoms worse.
- *Physical exhaustion or overexertion* is another common trigger, particularly for autoimmune flares, as it taxes the body's ability to regulate inflammation.

Understanding the factors that worsen EBV and autoimmune conditions provides insight into how these complex conditions interact with everyday life. Stress, gut health, diet, and environmental exposures are just a few of the triggers that can affect immune function, highlighting the importance of being mindful of how these elements influence overall health.

Supporting Your Immune System When Living with EBV & Autoimmune Disease

Living with Epstein-Barr Virus (EBV) and autoimmune diseases presents unique challenges, particularly when it comes to managing symptoms and maintaining overall health. This chapter focuses on objective insights into strategies that may support the immune system and reduce the burden of these conditions.

Here, we explore how factors like inflammation, nutrition, rest, and supplements may play a role in health management without prescribing specific steps.

How to Reduce Inflammation and Minimize Symptom Flares

Inflammation is a key factor in both EBV and autoimmune diseases, as it contributes to many of the common symptoms like pain, fatigue, and swelling. Understanding how inflammation works can provide insight into why flare-ups occur.

The Body and Immune System in Overdrive

Inflammation is the body's natural response to injury or infection, but when it becomes chronic, it can harm the body's own tissues. Both EBV reactivation and autoimmunity are linked to persistent inflammation, which may explain why some people experience flares of fatigue or pain during certain periods.

Triggers Worsening Inflammation

Inflammation often worsens due to external factors like stress, diet choices, and environmental irritants (explored earlier in this guide). Internal factors may also include an overproduction of proteins and molecules that activate the immune system, even during inactive phases of illness. This overactivity can result in flares, where symptoms suddenly worsen and then later subside.

Finding ways to calm and balance the immune system can help reduce inflammation, though everyone experiences this differently depending on their unique condition and triggers.

The Role of Nutrition in Managing EBV and Autoimmunity

The relationship between what you consume and how your immune system responds is a profound one. Nutrition doesn't just fuel the body; it affects how immune cells function, how inflammation develops, and how the body defends itself during infections and flares.

Anti-Inflammatory Nutrients

Certain foods contain compounds that are naturally anti-inflammatory. These foods may influence how the immune system behaves, especially in the long term. While not every type of food will affect all individuals the same way, diets rich in nutrient-dense vegetables, lean proteins, and healthy fats are commonly associated with better overall health.

Examples of nutrients linked to immune health include:

- *Omega-3 fatty acids*, often found in fish or certain seeds, support a balanced immune response.
- *Vitamins, such as C, D, and E*, play roles in reducing inflammation or boosting immune cell efficiency.
- *Zinc* is an essential mineral that helps immune cells combat viruses.

Understanding which dietary patterns align with reducing inflammation and supporting immune activity may be beneficial in guiding choices about what to eat. Patterns like excessive sugar or low nutrient intake can contribute to the opposite effect and potentially worsen symptoms.

Hydration and Immune Function

Staying hydrated is also an important aspect of supporting overall immune system health. Water plays a role in transporting nutrients to cells and removing waste materials, both of which are vital for maintaining a balanced immune response.

The Importance of Rest, Gentle Movement, and Mindfulness

Taking care of the immune system involves more than diet; it's also influenced by how you rest and move. This is especially true for individuals managing chronic conditions like EBV or autoimmune diseases, where overexertion or lack of rest can lead to setbacks.

Rest and Recovery

The body requires downtime to repair itself, which is why proper rest is critical. Sleep, in particular, has a direct effect on immune regulation. Poor sleep has been shown to increase cytokines, molecules involved in inflammation. Chronic lack of rest may make the body more vulnerable to viral reactivation and worsen autoimmune symptoms.

Gentle Physical Activity

While intense exercise may not always be appropriate during flares, gentle movement can have a positive impact on physical and emotional health. Activities like walking, stretching, or yoga may help maintain muscle strength, improve circulation, and even reduce stress levels, all of which can indirectly support the immune system.

The key is balance. Overexertion can lead to fatigue or worsen inflammation, so it's important to adapt activity levels to how the body feels on a particular day.

Mindfulness and Its Impact on Health

Mindfulness practices, such as meditation or deep breathing, have been shown to positively affect stress levels, which, as mentioned earlier, directly impact immune function. By reducing stress hormones like cortisol, mindfulness techniques may help improve overall well-being and contribute to better immune regulation.

Should You Take Supplements? What the Science Says

Supplements are often discussed as tools for supporting immune health, particularly in the context of deficiencies or unique needs during illness. However, it's important to look at what science says about their role in managing EBV or autoimmune diseases.

Supplements and Immune Support

Some supplements have been studied for their potential role in immune health. For instance, vitamin D is closely linked to immune regulation and may play a role for individuals who have low levels.

Zinc, vitamin C, and certain herbal extracts have also been examined for their possible effects on reducing inflammation or enhancing immune activity. However, not all findings are conclusive, and supplements rarely offer a one-size-fits-all solution.

Risks of Supplement Use

It's worth noting that supplements, especially in high doses, can have side effects or interact with medications commonly prescribed for autoimmune diseases. For instance, excessive vitamin D can lead to calcium buildup, and too much zinc can interfere with other mineral absorption in the body.

Questions of Effectiveness

While supplements may be useful under specific conditions, they are generally better at supporting general health or addressing deficiencies than directly preventing EBV reactivation or autoimmune flares. Reviewing any supplement use with a healthcare provider is essential to understand what's appropriate for an individual's specific circumstances.

Supporting the immune system when managing EBV and autoimmune diseases involves understanding the interplay between factors like inflammation, nutrition, physical activity, and rest. While no single solution exists, maintaining awareness of these influences allows for better management and a more balanced approach to health.

Navigating Medical & Holistic Approaches

Managing Epstein-Barr Virus (EBV) and autoimmune diseases can feel overwhelming, especially when trying to decide which medical or holistic approaches might be most helpful. Both conventional medicine and holistic practices offer valuable perspectives, and many people find that combining these approaches can provide a more comprehensive pathway to health.

This chapter explores what conventional medicine says about these conditions, introduces holistic options, highlights important blood tests to consider, and examines how integrative health practitioners may support your care.

What Conventional Medicine Says About EBV & Autoimmune Disease

Conventional medicine takes a structured, evidence-based approach to diagnosing and treating EBV and autoimmune diseases. While these systems of care often treat each condition separately, there is increasing recognition of their potential overlap.

EBV in Conventional Medicine

For most people, EBV is considered a dormant virus after the initial infection. Conventional doctors typically address EBV reactivation, such as in mononucleosis, by managing symptoms like fatigue, fever, and sore throat. Antiviral medications, while not commonly prescribed for mild EBV cases, might be considered for severe or chronic reactivation in immunocompromised individuals.

EBV's link to autoimmune diseases isn't fully understood, but ongoing research continues to explore how the virus might influence immune dysfunction. Most therapies for EBV in conventional settings focus on minimizing complications rather than eliminating the virus itself, which remains dormant in the body.

Autoimmune Diseases in Conventional Medicine

Autoimmune diseases are typically managed with treatments that aim to reduce inflammation and suppress an overactive immune response. Common therapies include:

- *Anti-inflammatory drugs* to control inflammation.
- *Immunosuppressants* to limit immune system overactivity.
- *Corticosteroids* to address acute flare-ups.

- ***Biologic drugs*** for targeted treatments in specific conditions like rheumatoid arthritis or lupus.

Conventional medicine provides critical tools for controlling autoimmune symptoms. However, these therapies generally focus on managing the condition rather than addressing root causes like potential viral triggers, including EBV.

Alternative & Holistic Approaches to Managing EBV

Holistic and alternative medicine often aims to support overall well-being while addressing possible underlying triggers of health issues. These approaches focus on strengthening the immune system, improving gut health, and reducing inflammation naturally.

Holistic Perspectives on EBV

Many holistic practitioners see EBV as a potential contributor to chronic health concerns. Their strategies often focus on creating an environment in the body that makes it harder for the virus to reactivate.

This might involve recommending lifestyle changes, stress management techniques, and nutritional support aimed at supporting immune balance. Some holistic approaches also explore natural remedies, such as herbal antivirals, though scientific research is still ongoing in this area.

Supporting Autoimmune Conditions Holistically

For autoimmune diseases, holistic approaches often center on reducing systemic inflammation and addressing triggers like diet, stress, and environmental toxins. Techniques like acupuncture, meditation, and anti-inflammatory diets are often incorporated with the goal of improving quality of life and minimizing symptom flares.

It's important to note that holistic approaches are generally used as a complement to conventional care and should be undertaken with a clear understanding of their potential benefits and limitations.

Blood Tests and Markers to Request from Your Doctor

Whether investigating EBV reactivation, an autoimmune condition, or both, certain blood tests can provide valuable insights. These tests help pinpoint what might be happening inside the body, offering clues to guide diagnosis and treatment options.

Tests for EBV

To determine whether EBV is active in the body, doctors may order tests to measure specific antibodies:

- *VCA-IgM (Viral Capsid Antigen-IgM):* Indicates a current or recent EBV infection.

- *VCA-IgG (Viral Capsid Antigen-IgG):* Shows past infection and immunity.
- *EA-D (Early Antigen-D):* This may indicate active EBV replication.
- *EBNA (Epstein-Barr Nuclear Antigen):* Usually appears after the acute phase and suggests past infection.

These markers can help confirm whether EBV reactivation might be contributing to symptoms, but their interpretation should always be discussed with a healthcare provider.

Tests for Autoimmune Conditions

Autoimmune conditions often require testing for specific markers to confirm a diagnosis or monitor disease activity. Common autoimmune-related tests include:

- *Antinuclear Antibodies (ANA):* Detects autoimmune activity in conditions like lupus.
- *Rheumatoid Factor (RF):* Used to diagnose rheumatoid arthritis.
- *Thyroid Antibodies:* Specific to Hashimoto's thyroiditis or Graves' disease.
- *C-reactive Protein (CRP) and Erythrocyte Sedimentation Rate (ESR):* Measure inflammation levels.

Working with a healthcare provider to order and interpret these tests allows for a more accurate picture of what might be causing symptoms.

Working with an Integrative Health Practitioner

Integrative health practitioners aim to combine the strengths of both conventional and holistic medicine. Their approach is designed to address the whole person, looking for underlying causes of illness while also managing symptoms effectively.

The Role of an Integrative Practitioner

Integrative health practitioners often work closely with their patients to develop personalized care plans. These may include:

- Collaborative efforts with conventional doctors to ensure appropriate medical treatments are in place.
- Recommendations for diet, lifestyle changes, or stress management to address root causes.
- Use of evidence-informed natural therapies to complement medical care.

How They Support Long-Term Wellness

Rather than focusing solely on individual symptoms, integrative practitioners try to understand how various factors such as stress, environmental triggers, and gut health contribute to a person's overall condition. They aim to create a tailored approach that aligns with a person's specific needs and goals.

It's worth mentioning that when working with holistic or integrative health practitioners, it's essential to choose a professional who is well-trained and communicates openly with other members of your healthcare team.

Both conventional and holistic treatments offer unique advantages when it comes to managing EBV and autoimmune diseases. By understanding their roles and tools—from blood tests to lifestyle changes and beyond—you can make more informed decisions about your care. Whether pursuing medical treatments, exploring holistic options, or working with an integrative practitioner, the most important step is to find what works best for your health and circumstances.

The next chapter will take a closer look at how to create a balanced approach that empowers you to live well despite the challenges of EBV and autoimmune diseases.

Long-Term Strategies for Managing EBV & Autoimmune Symptoms

Managing Epstein-Barr Virus (EBV) and autoimmune symptoms often requires a long-term approach that considers various aspects of health and daily life. While treatments may address acute symptoms, many people living with these conditions benefit from strategies focused on maintaining balance and reducing triggers.

This chapter explores several key areas to consider when managing EBV and autoimmune disease over time. These include lifestyle adjustments, prevention of EBV reactivation, emotional health, and creating individualized health plans.

Lifestyle Adjustments That Reduce Autoimmune Flares

For individuals managing autoimmune conditions, particularly those with links to Epstein-Barr Virus (EBV), lifestyle choices can significantly affect how often and how severe symptoms arise. Autoimmune flares often result when the immune system becomes excessively active, leading to inflammation and other uncomfortable symptoms.

EBV reactivation can further complicate matters by stressing the immune system. By focusing on certain aspects of daily life, people can create a supportive environment for their bodies, potentially reducing the frequency and intensity of flares.

Here are some key lifestyle adjustments to consider, each explained in detail for better understanding.

1. **The Role of Nutrition**

    Nutrition plays a crucial role in maintaining overall health and immune function. A diet that supports the immune system may help reduce inflammation, a common factor in both autoimmune activity and EBV symptoms.

    <u>Choosing Nutrient-Rich Foods</u>

    Whole, unprocessed foods are often ideal for supporting immune health. Fruits, vegetables, nuts, seeds, whole grains, and lean proteins provide essential vitamins, minerals, and antioxidants. For example:

    - ***Colorful vegetables like spinach and bell peppers*** are packed with vitamins A and C, which help protect cells and repair damaged tissues.

- ***Fatty fish such as salmon*** provide omega-3 fatty acids, which have anti-inflammatory properties.
- ***Nuts and seeds***, such as almonds and flaxseeds, supply nutrients like magnesium and zinc, which are important for immune regulation.

Reducing Pro-Inflammatory Foods

On the other hand, certain foods can contribute to higher inflammation levels. Diets that include large amounts of processed foods, refined sugars, trans fats, and saturated fats have been linked to an increase in inflammatory markers. For instance:

- Regular consumption of sugary beverages or snacks can lead to spikes in blood sugar and may irritate systems already prone to inflammation.
- Foods like fried fast food or heavily processed packaged meals often contain unhealthy fats or additives.

Identifying Personal Triggers

Because autoimmune responses vary widely between individuals, some may notice specific foods worsen their symptoms. For example, gluten may be a trigger for individuals with celiac disease or other inflammatory disorders. Paying close attention to how the body reacts after eating certain foods can help guide personal dietary adjustments.

2. **Physical Activity and Movement**

Physical activity can have a profound effect on both EBV-related fatigue and symptoms of autoimmune diseases. However, striking the right balance between movement and rest is essential for people with chronic conditions.

Benefits of Regular Movement

Regular movement benefits the immune system and promotes overall circulation. It can also help alleviate stiffness, muscle tension, and joint pain often associated with autoimmune diseases. Low-impact activities such as walking, swimming, or yoga are generally well-tolerated and provide the following advantages:

- *Improved circulation* supports oxygen and nutrient delivery to tissues.
- *Reduction in stiffness* helps maintain joint mobility, particularly in conditions like rheumatoid arthritis.
- *Energy stabilization* may occur as short exercises counteract feelings of sluggishness or fatigue.

Avoiding Overexertion

While regular movement is beneficial, overdoing it can cause harm, especially for those already dealing with fatigue or flare-ups. High-intensity workouts or extended exercise sessions may strain the body rather than energize it. It's important to pace physical activity and listen to the body's signals, particularly during periods of low energy or heightened symptoms.

Examples of Gentle Exercises

Simple exercises can be incorporated into daily routines without excessive strain. Suggestions include:

- ***Stretching or yoga*** to alleviate tightness and promote relaxation.
- ***Walking for 10–20 minutes*** to boost circulation without overexerting the system.
- ***Swimming or water aerobics*** to provide joint-friendly resistance that minimizes impact.

3. **Sleep and Rest**

    Sleep is one of the body's most powerful tools for repair and immune regulation. A lack of restorative sleep can exacerbate both autoimmune flares and EBV reactivation, highlighting the importance of prioritizing rest.

    ### How Sleep Impacts Health

Quality sleep allows the body to produce immune cells that fight infections and repair damaged tissues. On the other hand, poor sleep can reduce the production of protective cytokines, which the immune system uses to combat stress and illness. Chronic sleep disruptions may also increase levels of inflammation, complicating autoimmune conditions.

Establishing a Sleep Routine

Creating a consistent sleep routine can help individuals achieve better quality rest. This includes:

- Going to bed and waking up at the same time daily, even on weekends.
- Avoid stimulants such as caffeine at least six hours before bedtime.
- Limiting exposure to screens (phones, TVs, tablets) close to bedtime, as blue light can hinder the production of melatonin, a hormone essential for sleep.

Relaxation Techniques for Better Sleep

People managing autoimmune or EBV-related fatigue often benefit from strategies to calm the mind before bed. Relaxation techniques may include:

- *Deep breathing exercises*, slow heart rate and prepare the body for rest.

- ***Reading a book or listening to calming music*** to transition into a more peaceful state.
- Using ***meditation or guided imagery*** to reduce stress and quiet racing thoughts.

4. **Stress Management**

   Stress is a well-known trigger for both autoimmune flares and EBV reactivation. Emotional or physical stress causes the release of cortisol, a hormone that, when elevated, can suppress immune function and increase inflammation.

   The Effects of Chronic Stress

   When stress becomes chronic, it takes a toll on the immune system. High cortisol levels impair the immune response, making the body less able to regulate itself or keep dormant viruses like EBV in check. Prolonged stress may also negatively affect sleep, digestion, and energy levels, compounding the challenges faced by individuals with autoimmune conditions.

   Incorporating Stress-Reduction Activities

   Stress management practices provide an opportunity to alleviate some of the emotional and physical effects of chronic stress. Some effective methods include:

- ***Mindfulness and meditation*** to focus on the present moment and reduce anxiety.
- ***Journaling*** as a form of emotional release and reflection.
- ***Spending time in nature***, such as taking a walk in a park, to experience calming surroundings.

Personalizing Stress Management

What works for one person may not work for another. It's important to explore different techniques and identify which is most effective in reducing stress levels. For instance, one person might find yoga relaxing, while another prefers gardening or painting as a creative outlet.

While no single lifestyle adjustment can completely prevent autoimmune flares or eliminate the challenges posed by EBV, combining these strategies creates a holistic approach to symptom management.

Paying attention to nutrition, physical activity, sleep, and stress allows the body to function at its best, potentially decreasing the effects of these conditions over time. By observing and listening to their body's responses, individuals can develop a routine that promotes better resilience and overall well-being.

How to Prevent EBV Reactivation in the Future

Epstein-Barr Virus (EBV) is known for its ability to lie dormant in the body after the initial infection and reappear under certain conditions. Reactivation of EBV can lead to symptoms that interfere with daily life and may even worsen existing health issues.

While it's impossible to completely eliminate the virus once it's in the body, there are ways to lower the likelihood of its reactivation. This involves understanding the factors that contribute to reactivation and taking practical steps to support immunity and reduce potential triggers.

1. **Supporting Immune Health**

    A strong and balanced immune system plays a critical role in keeping EBV dormant. When the immune system functions optimally, it's better equipped to suppress EBV activity and prevent the virus from reactivating.

    The Importance of Balanced Nutrition

    Food provides the building blocks your body needs to maintain a healthy immune system. Eating a balanced diet full of nutrient-dense, whole foods can help support immune health. Nutrients particularly beneficial for immunity include:

- *Vitamin C*: Found in oranges, strawberries, broccoli, and bell peppers, it helps protect cells and promotes the production of infection-fighting white blood cells.
- *Vitamin D*: Essential for immune regulation, this nutrient is found in fatty fish, fortified foods, and can also be absorbed through sunlight exposure. Many people with low vitamin D levels may benefit from addressing this deficiency to improve immune function.
- *Zinc*: Found in nuts, seeds, beans, and meat, zinc supports processes that help repair tissues and produce immune cells.
- *Antioxidants* (like those in berries, spinach, and green tea): These neutralize the free radicals that can damage cells.

Staying hydrated, avoiding excessive intake of processed or sugary foods, and ensuring an adequate variety of nutrients are also key aspects of a healthy diet.

Incorporating Physical Activity

Regular physical activity supports both the cardiovascular and immune systems, helping to improve overall resilience. Moderate-intensity exercises like brisk walking, stretching, cycling, or yoga are particularly beneficial because:

- They increase circulation, which helps immune cells travel throughout the body more efficiently.
- Lower-intensity workouts are less likely than intense, vigorous routines to cause overexertion, which can stress the immune system.

The goal is to find a sustainable routine. Short, consistent sessions of activity may be more effective for those managing chronic fatigue or other symptoms associated with EBV or autoimmune conditions.

Quality Sleep and Rest

Sleep is when the body works to repair and restore itself, and it's vital for immune balance. Chronic sleep deprivation has been linked to weakened immunity, leaving the body more vulnerable to viral reactivation. To establish healthier sleep habits:

- Aim for **seven to nine hours** of sleep per night.
- Stick to a consistent sleep schedule, even on weekends.
- Create a calming bedtime routine, such as reading or meditating, to signal to your brain that it's time to wind down.

If poor sleep persists due to other issues like insomnia, addressing these through relaxation techniques or discussing options with a healthcare provider may help prevent chronic sleep deprivation from overwhelming the immune system.

Avoiding Harmful Habits

Certain behaviors may negatively impact immune regulation, making EBV reactivation more likely. Smoking, for example, damages the respiratory system and suppresses immune function. Similarly, heavy alcohol consumption can reduce the body's ability to fight infections. Reducing or avoiding these habits entirely can promote long-term immune stability.

2. **Avoiding Known Triggers**

Understanding the factors that can lead to EBV reactivation is key to managing potential threats. While not all triggers can be avoided completely, identifying and reducing personal risk factors can help.

Reducing Stress

Stress is one of the most common triggers of EBV reactivation. When stress builds up, the body produces higher levels of cortisol, a stress hormone that can suppress the immune system temporarily. To minimize stress:

- Practice mindfulness techniques, such as deep breathing, that help calm the mind and body.

- Include relaxation exercises like yoga or tai chi in your routine.
- Make time for hobbies and activities that relax or bring joy.

For those exposed to high levels of chronic stress, professional support, such as counseling or therapy, can make the task of managing stress feel more achievable.

Minimizing Illness and Physical Strain

Other illnesses, whether mild infections like the flu or chronic conditions requiring significant recovery, can tax the immune system. This increases the chances of EBV reactivation, as the immune system may struggle to keep the virus suppressed when overburdened. Simple measures to reduce the risk of illness include:

- **Washing hands frequently** to prevent the spread of germs.
- **Staying up to date on vaccinations**, such as for seasonal flu, which can decrease the risk of secondary infections.

Additionally, being mindful of physical overexertion and allowing enough time for rest during illnesses or recovery periods can prevent excessive immune stress.

Environmental and Chemical Exposures

While specific environmental toxins are difficult to measure, there is evidence that pollutants and certain harmful chemicals may contribute to immune disturbance. This includes frequent exposure to pesticides, certain industrial chemicals, or heavy metals. Reducing contact with these substances when possible, such as through regular hand washing, proper ventilation indoors, or limiting processed and packaged products exposed to toxins, may support immune balance.

Individualized Triggers

While stress, illness, and environmental factors are common triggers, individual sensitivities may also play a role. For example, hormonal imbalances during puberty, pregnancy, or menopause may be associated with heightened viral activity for some. Tracking triggers through a journal or health app may help individuals identify patterns and environments that affect their symptoms.

3. **Monitoring and Early Intervention**

Recognizing the early warning signs of EBV reactivation can help individuals respond more effectively, potentially reducing flare severity or duration. While self-monitoring isn't about self-diagnosis, it's a way to stay informed about changes in your body.

Observing Symptoms

Early symptoms of reactivation often mimic mild flu-like conditions but may also include signs such as:

- Persistent or extreme fatigue that doesn't improve with rest
- Swollen or tender lymph nodes, particularly in the neck or armpits
- Low-grade fever or recurring sore throat
- Vague muscle aches or headaches

Recording these symptoms when they occur can provide useful data points to share with healthcare providers. Patterns may emerge, such as symptom flare-ups during high-stress periods.

Seeking Professional Guidance

If symptoms of EBV reactivation become frequent or severe, consulting a healthcare professional may help in managing the condition. While there is no direct cure for EBV, supportive care to reduce inflammation, manage fatigue, and stabilize the immune reaction may improve quality of life.

Staying Proactive

Taking preventive steps, even during periods of dormancy, contributes to long-term management. For example, continuing stress reduction, exercise, and balanced nutrition can provide the body with a better baseline to fight reactivation when it arises.

While EBV cannot be fully eliminated from the body, many aspects of life can be adjusted to reduce the risk of reactivation. By focusing on immune health, minimizing exposure to personal triggers, and being attentive to early warning signs, individuals can take an active role in keeping EBV in check. It's the combination of these steps, applied consistently over time, that helps create a stronger foundation to maintain dormancy and improve overall well-being.

Emotional and Mental Health: Coping with a Chronic Condition

Living with a chronic condition like EBV-related autoimmune disease often extends beyond physical symptoms. Emotional and mental health challenges, such as anxiety, depression, or frustration, can become part of the daily experience. It's important to recognize these challenges and explore ways to adapt.

1. **The Emotional Toll of Chronic Illness**

    Feeling overwhelmed or discouraged is a common response to navigating an unpredictable condition.

Fluctuations in symptoms can disrupt daily routines, interfere with plans, and impact personal and professional relationships. Accepting the need for ongoing adjustments may be emotionally taxing, adding to the burden of physical discomfort.

2. Developing Resilience

Building mental resilience can be an important part of coping with chronic illness. Resilience doesn't mean avoiding negative emotions but rather finding ways to work through them and maintain perspective.

For some, this process includes seeking professional counseling or therapy. Cognitive-behavioral therapy (CBT) and other therapeutic approaches may be helpful in reframing challenges and fostering emotional adaptability.

3. Connecting with Community

Many individuals find shared understanding and encouragement through support groups or online communities. Hearing from others with shared experiences can provide a sense of belonging and lessen feelings of isolation. Support groups often serve as spaces where people exchange coping strategies or just listen, offering validation and camaraderie.

4. **The Importance of Self-Acceptance**

   Self-acceptance involves acknowledging both limitations and strengths. It includes understanding that some days may be harder than others and that seeking help when needed is not a sign of failure. Practicing self-compassion may assist individuals in navigating the ups and downs of living with a chronic condition.

Creating a Personalized Health Plan That Works for You

When living with a condition as complex as EBV-related autoimmune disease, no single approach works for everyone. A personalized health plan that accounts for individual needs, symptoms, and triggers can serve as a valuable tool for long-term management.

1. **Assessing Individual Needs**

   The first step in creating a personalized health plan is understanding one's specific condition and challenges. Factors like medical history, current symptoms, and lifestyle can all inform the plan. Working with health professionals to identify key goals, such as reducing symptom severity or maintaining energy levels, can provide clarity.

2. **Tracking Symptoms and Patterns**

   Keeping a health journal is one way to document patterns and potential triggers. Detailed notes about dietary choices, activity levels, stress, and symptoms may help individuals identify what worsens their condition or promote improvement. Over time, this information becomes a reference for making informed adjustments.

3. **Combining Medical and Holistic Approaches**

   A collaborative approach to care, involving both conventional and holistic practices, may offer more comprehensive support. Under the guidance of health practitioners, individuals might explore complementary strategies, such as acupuncture or dietary modifications, alongside medical treatments like medications or therapies for autoimmune conditions. The key is finding the right balance for each person's unique needs.

4. **Setting Reasonable Goals**

   For those managing EBV and autoimmune disease, progress may be gradual. Creating small, actionable goals rather than focusing on complete symptom elimination may be more realistic. Goals might include improving sleep quality, reducing the frequency of flares, or maintaining energy for specific activities.

Every small step can contribute to a greater sense of control and achievement.

5. **Maintaining Flexibility**

    Because chronic conditions often evolve, health plans should remain adaptable. Regular check-ins with healthcare providers and updates to the plan may help ensure it continues to meet changing needs and circumstances.

Long-term management of EBV and autoimmune symptoms requires a multifaceted approach. By making targeted lifestyle adjustments, working to prevent EBV reactivation, addressing mental and emotional health, and crafting individualized health plans, individuals can create a framework to support their overall well-being. While challenges may persist, developing strategies that align with personal needs and goals provides a pathway to greater stability and quality of life.

Conclusion

Managing a chronic condition such as EBV or an autoimmune disease requires an ongoing commitment to understanding your body, recognizing patterns, and implementing strategies that promote long-term well-being. While the path to feeling better is rarely straightforward, equipping yourself with knowledge and applying it progressively can lead to meaningful improvements in your quality of life. Adopting a mindset of exploration and patience is key, as recovery often unfolds gradually rather than in leaps.

Healing should be viewed as a continuous process, rather than an endpoint. Each individual's experience with health is unique, requiring trial and adjustment to determine what works best. For example, paying attention to daily habits, such as ensuring adequate sleep or incorporating nourishing meals into your routine, can lay a foundation for improvement.

These incremental actions, although seemingly small, contribute to building a structure of better health over time.

By framing healing as a collective result of these efforts, rather than expecting quick resolutions, you can align your focus on steady progress and reduce frustration.

Understanding and tracking symptoms is another fundamental step in managing your condition. Paying attention to how your body responds to various factors, such as certain foods or environmental changes, can reveal patterns.

Maintaining a record of your experiences, whether through a journal or a mobile app, provides a clearer picture of how symptoms evolve. This can help you identify correlations between your activities and how you feel; for example, you might notice worsening fatigue after exposure to stress or specific dietary choices.

Such insights not only guide personal decisions but also enhance communication with healthcare providers. Describing well-documented trends during medical appointments allows for a more personalized and effective treatment strategy.

Accessing external support and resources also plays a critical role in successfully navigating life with chronic conditions. The guidance of healthcare professionals, whether general practitioners, specialists, or integrative health practitioners, offers medically sound advice tailored to your case. Educational resources, such as scientifically credible articles, podcasts, or webinars, deepen your understanding of the relationship between EBV and autoimmune disorders.

Online communities and local support groups can provide additional perspectives and affirmations, as they connect you to others who share similar experiences. Engaging with these networks not only offers practical tips but also combats the emotional strain of managing long-term conditions, helping you feel less isolated.

Additionally, mental well-being is an integral piece of overall health management. Chronic illnesses often bring emotional challenges, requiring equal attention to psychological and emotional health. Many individuals benefit from activities that reduce stress, such as mindfulness exercises, counseling, or participating in creative outlets. Taking steps to foster mental and emotional resilience enhances your capacity to cope with the unpredictable nature of chronic conditions.

An empowered approach involves actively incorporating what you learn into your lifestyle. This can mean prioritizing consistent efforts, such as creating a space for relaxation, making mindful dietary changes, or reflecting on your daily experiences.

Over time, these efforts, strengthened by support systems and professional guidance, can help establish a sense of control over both immediate and long-term health outcomes. Facing these challenges with an adaptable and informed mindset lays the groundwork for living in harmony with your condition.

FAQs

What is Epstein-Barr Virus (EBV), and how is it connected to autoimmune diseases?

EBV is a member of the herpesvirus family that remains dormant in most people after infection. Research suggests that EBV may contribute to the development of autoimmune diseases by altering immune system responses or triggering inflammation that leads to immune system malfunction.

Can EBV cause autoimmune diseases directly?

While EBV alone does not directly cause autoimmune diseases, it is believed to act as a trigger in some individuals with genetic or environmental predispositions. For example, EBV may play a role in conditions like multiple sclerosis (MS), lupus, and rheumatoid arthritis.

What symptoms might indicate a connection between EBV and an autoimmune condition?

Symptoms can overlap between EBV and autoimmune diseases, including chronic fatigue, joint pain, swollen lymph nodes, low-grade fever, and muscle aches. Persistent or recurring symptoms could suggest autoimmune involvement or EBV reactivation and warrant medical evaluation.

What are the key triggers for EBV reactivation, and do they worsen autoimmune symptoms?

EBV can reactivate due to factors like stress, illness, hormonal changes, or immune suppression. Reactivation may lead to inflammation and exacerbate symptoms in people already managing autoimmune diseases, such as increased fatigue or joint discomfort.

How can someone distinguish EBV symptoms from autoimmune flare-ups?

EBV symptoms often fluctuate and tend to align with viral reactivation, such as sore throat or swollen lymph nodes. Autoimmune flare-ups may be more chronic and involve inflammation-specific symptoms like joint swelling or organ involvement. Tracking symptoms over time can provide clues to their origin.

What lifestyle adjustments can help manage EBV-related symptoms and reduce autoimmune flares?

Supporting immune health by maintaining a nutrient-rich diet, engaging in moderate exercise, prioritizing quality sleep, and managing stress may help reduce the impact of both EBV and autoimmune conditions. Avoiding known triggers such as environmental toxins or overexertion is also beneficial.

Is it possible to completely cure EBV or prevent its reactivation?

Currently, there is no cure for EBV, as the virus remains dormant in the body for life. However, understanding and addressing reactivation triggers, while supporting overall immune health, can significantly reduce the risk of symptoms and minimize their severity.

References and Helpful Links

Epstein-Barr virus. (2025, January 3). Cleveland Clinic. https://my.clevelandclinic.org/health/diseases/23469-epstein-barr-virus

Steinman, L., MD, Obeidat, A., MD PhD, Frcpc, A. B. M., & Mph, B. a. B. M. (2022, July 21). The role of Epstein-Barr virus in autoimmune diseases. Neurology Live. https://www.neurologylive.com/view/the-role-of-epstein-barr-virus-in-autoimmune-diseases

Nierengarten, M. B. (2023, September 28). Study implicates Epstein-Barr virus in 7 autoimmune diseases - The rheumatologist. The Rheumatologist. https://www.the-rheumatologist.org/article/study-implicates-epstein-barr-virus-in-7-autoimmune-diseases/

Dellwo, A. (2023, November 16). Autoimmune diseases associated with Epstein-Barr virus. Verywell Health. https://www.verywellhealth.com/is-epstein-barr-linked-to-autoimmune-disease-4165847

Seladi-Schulman, J., PhD. (2023, May 25). Everything you need to know about Epstein-Barr virus. Healthline. https://www.healthline.com/health/epstein-barr-virus

About Epstein-Barr virus (EBV). (2024, May 9). Epstein-Barr Virus and Infectious Mononucleosis. https://www.cdc.gov/epstein-barr/about/index.html#:~:text=There%20is%20no%20specific%20treatment,Getting%20plenty%20of%20rest

Laboratory testing for Epstein-Barr virus (EBV). (2024, April 10). Epstein-Barr Virus and Infectious Mononucleosis. https://www.cdc.gov/epstein-barr/php/laboratories/index.html#:~:text=Viral%20capsid%20antigen%20(VCA),rest%20of%20a%20person's%20life.

www.ingramcontent.com/pod-product-compliance
Lightning Source LLC
LaVergne TN
LVHW012054070526
838201LV00083B/4580